trotman

REAL LIFE ISSUES:
STRESS

Rozina Breen

Real Life Issues: Stress
This first edition published in 2004 by Trotman and Company Ltd
2 The Green, Richmond, Surrey TW9 1PL

Editorial and Publishing Team
Author Rozina Breen
Editorial Mina Patria, Editorial Director; Rachel Lockhart, Commissioning Editor;
Anya Wilson, Managing Editor; Bianca Knights, Assistant Editor
Production Ken Ruskin, Head of Pre-press and Production;
James Rudge, Production Artworker
Sales and Marketing Deborah Jones, Head of Sales and Marketing
Advertising Tom Lee, Commercial Director
Managing Director Toby Trotman

Designed by XAB

British Library Cataloguing in Publication Data
A catalogue record for this book is available from the British Library

ISBN 0 85660 989 7

Typeset by Tradespools Publishing Solutions
Printed and bound in Great Britain by
Cromwell Press, Trowbridge, Wiltshire

CONTENTS:

'Once you learn to recognise the symptoms of stress, you can follow the advice on how to beat it.'

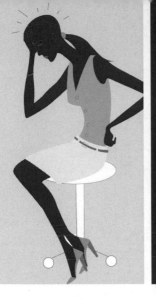

REAL LIFE ISSUES:
Stress

ABOUT THE AUTHOR

Rozina Breen worked as a senior producer for the BBC's Current Affairs unit in London until very recently. She has worked on a variety of programmes for BBC1, BBC2, Radio 4 and also 5 Live. She studied English and Drama at University College of Wales, Aberystwyth and also obtained a Master's degree from the University of Leeds. When she's not writing or making radio programmes, she paints by commission. She lives in Yorkshire with her husband and three young children.

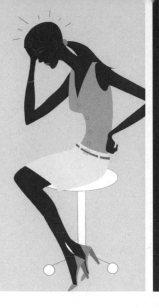

REAL LIFE ISSUES:
Stress

ACKNOWLEDGEMENTS

Many thanks to the following for their invaluable help and information: Kidscape; the Science Museum; BBC Radio 1; KidsHealth and The Nemours Foundation; Gladeana McMahon at the Centre for Stress Management; Department of Health; Young Minds; At Ease; Jane Kettle; Frances Hayes; Alice Leahy; Lauren Fox; Simran Hunjan; and Georgina Hughes.

David, Seamus, Jakey and Laily...and, as always, to Rumina.

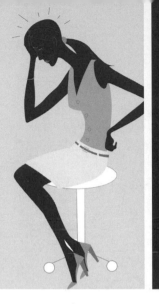

INTRODUCTION
Recognising the symptoms of stress

How often do you hear people say, 'this is really stressing me out'? These days, it seems, stress is just part and parcel of everyday life.

It's not surprising, really. Just think about how busy our lives have become. And there's so much pressure to get more things done even more quickly than ever before.

Stress doesn't just affect adults. Research has shown that toddlers as young as three can experience it. And you, too, are likely to be a victim of stress at one stage or another during your teenage years

FACT BOX

The Samaritans
The Samaritans take around five million calls a year – that's four times as many as they were taking 25 years ago.

There is pressure coming at you from teachers, expectations from the people who look after you, and even hassle from friends. You might have exams, homework, after-school clubs and loads of other things going on in your life that, at times, feel very hard to juggle.

Approximately two out of three of us feel stressed out at least once a month.

Samaritans

GREAT EXPECTATIONS

Adults tend to view the world of anyone under the age of 18 as happy and carefree. You might hear them say, 'you don't know you're born', or that their youth was the best time of their life. Things are very different now, though.

Society has never been more competitive than it is today and there's a heap of expectation placed on your shoulders. Achieving good results and fitting as much as possible into each day can all seem too much at times. And although whoever looks after you means well, their demands on you – to do well, for example – can add to the stress you feel. They expect the world from you, but let's face it, that's not easy to deliver.

For some, the stress is so uncontrollable that life seems unbearable. In fact, recent research shows that every hour three young people harm themselves (cutting their skin at times of stress, or taking an overdose, then calling 999) – that's double what it was 25 years ago.

The stress you feel comes from two opposite directions: outside and inside. Outside pressure comes from parents, carers, teachers and friends, for example. Inside pressure is the kind of pressure that we put on ourselves to do well. And that has a huge influence on the way we cope.

The reasons you get stressed won't just come from what's happening in your own life. There might be problems at work for your mum or dad or whoever looks after you, squabbles at home (about money, for instance), and arguments between family members. All these can make you feel anxious, but recognising stress can be hard because it's not as simple as diagnosing something physical like chickenpox or tonsillitis. There are signals, however, that can help you spot it.

THE SYMPTOMS OF STRESS

Do you:
- have problems sleeping?
- find it difficult to concentrate?
- prefer to spend time on your own?
- generally feel slightly unwell?
- suffer from frequent stomach-aches or headaches?

If you've answered 'yes' to two or more of these questions you could be suffering from stress.

REDUCING STRESS

Making sure you have enough time to relax is really important, and later on in the book you'll find some useful tips for doing just that. But there's also that phrase, 'a problem shared is a problem halved'. It might sound old-fashioned, but it's amazing how a simple conversation can make you more confident about the future and also help you feel in control again.

For many teenagers, talking to your mum or dad or whoever looks after you might not be an option. You might feel that they wouldn't really understand what you're going through. But there are other adults you could turn to: a teacher or a family friend, for example. Remember, you don't always have to take their advice!

And if talking to any adult seems completely out of the question, why not try talking to a friend? You can be pretty sure that they've had their own fair share of stress, and they might just have found a good method of getting through it.

Read on ...

There are all sorts of different ways of reducing stress – from planning what you eat to simple breathing exercises. This book will guide you through some different remedies. It will also outline some of the more common reasons for getting stressed, but remember: different things are stressful for different people. Once you learn to recognise the symptoms of stress, you can follow the advice on how to beat it. You might decide to follow every bit of advice, or you might just pick up one or two tips along the way; but even that will be a great start. One move forward can help you feel more in control of your life.

But first, to really get on top of something, you need to understand it. So it's a good idea to find out exactly what stress is and how it can affect your mental as well as your physical health.

CHAPTER ONE:

WHAT IS STRESS?
How you can tell if you're stressed

So you think you might be stressed? Identifying what's causing your anxiety will certainly help you overcome it. But understanding how stress affects both your mind and your body will help you begin to make sense of it all.

STRESSORS

A **stressor** is another name for the trigger that sets off your stress. These don't have to be big, traumatic events. Missing a bus or having to give a talk in front of your class can make you feel the emotions linked to stress – anger, frustration and worry, for example.

Stressors are divided into two types: internal and external. Each of these can be physical or psychological. So for example, pain is a **physical stressor** – and it's caused externally. But worrying about the way you look is an **internal stressor** that starts off psychologically – that's to say, the worry begins in your own mind.

Internal psychological stress can often be the most harmful because there is no easy solution. These stressors are anxieties about events

FACT BOX

*An age-old concept
The idea that the state of your mind can affect your health is nothing new. In fact, historians believe that Hippocrates, a doctor who lived around 5 BC, came up with the idea, and it's been going ever since.*

that may or may not happen, and as long as you're worrying about it, your body will be affected by the way you feel.

CHEMICAL REACTIONS

What exactly happens to your body when you get stressed?

When we find ourselves in stressful situations, our body responds with a biochemical reaction, producing hormones that have specific physical effects. That natural reaction is known as the **stress response** and it can be triggered by physical or emotional demands.

The stress response is a survival mechanism, an evolutionary adaptation that helped our ancestors cope in a world filled with life-threatening dangers … lions, tigers and bears, to name a few. Our body responds instinctively to danger by preparing us both physically and mentally for a challenge. A mixture of chemical messengers and hormones are released that make us more alert and provide us with a rush of energy.

The stress response has equipped us to cope brilliantly in challenging situations. Our ancestors survived because they had the physical and mental capabilities to run from, or fight with, anything that threatened them. OK, so lions might not be chasing you to school every morning, but modern life does present us with other hazards. Wouldn't you want to be able to run away as fast as you could if you thought you were in some kind of danger?

We make use of the stress response even when we're not feeling threatened. Take a race, for example. You won't die if you don't run fast enough. But the hormones and chemicals that pump around your body when you get stressed increase the amount of oxygen and energy getting to your muscles, making you run faster than you could if you were perfectly calm.

Getting stressed before an exam is also quite common, but did you know the stress response in that situation can actually make your mind sharper?

Strange though it sounds, stress can actually be quite rewarding. Adrenaline is one of the hormones released during the stress response, and no doubt you've heard the phrase 'adrenaline rush'. It's that buzz we get after asking someone out on a date, or finishing a set of exams, and it seems to make all that stressing worth it in the end.

FACT BOX

Sweaty palms? Shaky knees? Thumping heart? Adrenaline rush? That's your body's stress response doing its job.

Lots of people seek out adrenaline rushes by engineering stressful situations for themselves – ever watched a horror film, gone on a roller coaster or sky dived? The good thing about scaring yourself on a roller coaster, though, is that you know it's not going to last that long!

The problem with stress is when it goes on for a long time. It can have a bad effect on both your mind and your body. So dealing with bad stress as soon as you're able to recognise it is really important. Long-lasting (or chronic) stress can wear you out, make you feel exhausted and out of control. And it can also weaken your immune system, making you a prime target for bugs and ill health.

YOUR KIND OF STRESS

Everyone gets stressed by different things. What causes your anxieties might not bother your best friend at all.

As a nation, though, there are some things that stress us all more than others. A survey commissioned by the Samaritans in 2002 revealed that:
- the biggest stress for British 16–24-year-olds was university, college or school
- the next biggest cause of stress for young people was money, with one in four regularly getting stressed about their finances.

Experts say we all have different stress 'thresholds': that is to say, the point where the stress you experience starts to have a negative effect. For example, when you start to feel worried, scared and unable to deal with the situation. The threshold is the tipping point that leads you to start feeling out of control.

Someone with a low threshold can get very stressed by simple events, like being late or forgetting their keys. But for someone with a high threshold it would take something much bigger to stress them out – failing an exam or moving house are good examples.

Scientists have identified a series of different factors that can influence how badly you are affected by stress. Your age and sex can make a difference to the way you cope, but a big factor is your personality type.

Psychologists talk about two personality types when it comes to stress: A or B. People with **Type A personalities** are more likely to **rush**, to be **competitive** and to be **perfectionists**. They often attempt to do two or more things at once and feel guilty when they take time out to relax or do nothing, even if it's just for a couple of hours.

Type B personalities, on the other hand, are people who can be described as **'laid back'**. They are **easy-going**, able to work at a **reasonable pace** and can **relax** without feeling guilty.

Not surprisingly, Type A people are much more prone to stress than Type B people. Any minor event that disrupts their normal routine or gets in the way of their plans can upset a Type A person, while a Type B person is much more able to take things in their stride. They're better able to put things in perspective, thinking through how they are going to deal with a situation rather than just stressing over it as a Type A person would.

Type A or Type B?

The following two boxes outline some typical traits from each of the personality types A and B. They're not going to describe you exactly – you're probably a combination of descriptions in both lists – but one should stand out more than the other when it comes to describing what you're like.

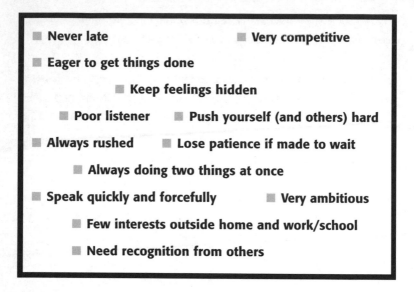

Figure 1 A Type personality traits

Or are you mostly these?

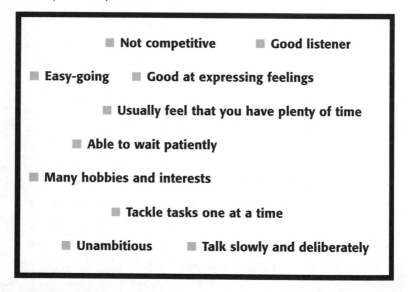

Figure 2 B Type personality traits

If you've got more ticks in the first box, then you're more likely to lean towards a Type A personality – but if you have more in common with the traits in the second box, you're more likely to have a Type B personality. If you had exactly the same number of ticks in each box, you'd put a marker halfway between the two personality types. The more As you tick, the further you move your marker to point A; and the more Bs you tick, the further you move your marker to point B.

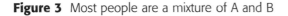

Type A ├ ─ ─ ─ ─ ─ ─ ─ ┼ ─ ─ ─ ─ ─ ─ ─ ─ ─ ─ ─ ─ ─ ┤ Type B

Figure 3 Most people are a mixture of A and B

In reality though, there is no absolute division between Type A and Type B personalities. People usually fall somewhere on a line linking the two, leaning more towards one type than the other. The closer you are to one personality type, the more likely it is that you will display the character traits of that type.

What researchers have found is that people who display more Type A characteristics have a higher risk of suffering from stress-related illnesses, such as high blood pressure and high cholesterol, than their Type B friends. They are also more inclined to turn to cigarettes and alcohol in order to help them deal with stress.

However, it is important to remember that you are not doomed! If you are edging towards the Type A end of the scale, it just means that you have to develop some effective de-stressing techniques and be vigilant about not letting yourself become overwhelmed.

TELLTALE SIGNS OF STRESS

Do you get spots, unexplained rashes, tummy cramps, diarrhoea, headaches? Are you constantly picking up bugs?

If so, you could be suffering from stress. Our bodies tend to reflect our emotional wellbeing. When we're stressed our immune system doesn't operate as well as it normally does, so it's easier to get ill and we also take longer to get better.

Although some people lose weight when they are stressed, more often than not we put weight on. That's because the balance of sugars and fats in our blood changes and we can start to crave salty, fatty and sugary foods.

A stressed person will find it hard to sleep, so you might start to feel tired and lack your usual energy.

TRY THE QUIZ

Everyone has problems with their mental health at some point or other – we may feel down, anxious or confused. .

One young person in five has mental health problems.
                                Young Minds mental health charity

But, just as with our physical health, there are ways to prevent some mental health problems taking over. And if you find yourself tipping the balance of your 'threshold' there are solutions to getting back on track.

The best thing to do is know what to look for and where to go for help if you need it. Just being aware of your feelings is a good way of beginning to stay on top of things.

QUIZ

In the last three months have you:

1. Felt very tired, run down or lost your appetite?
2. Found it difficult to concentrate or make decisions?
3. Felt strange or different, but have not been able to explain how or why?
4. Lost someone close to you due to a relationship break-up, moving house or someone dying?
5. Seen or heard things that other people have not?
6. Had headaches, backaches or stomach-aches that don't seem to go away?

Now add up your score. If you answered:
yes to question 1 score 1 point
yes to question 2 score 1 point
yes to question 3 score 2 points
yes to question 4 score 2 points
yes to question 5 score 3 points
yes to question 6 score 2 points.

If you scored 0–1 point:
You seem to be maintaining a good level of mental fitness – the challenge now is to keep it up. Keep checking your fitness levels. Be

aware as soon as your fitness level starts to go down. Just as with all forms of health, the sooner you deal with any problems, the more likely you are to make a full, lasting recovery. Email this quiz to family and friends. One in four of us will have problems with our mental health at some point in our lives, so no matter how fit the people you care about are right now, it's important they check their mental fitness regularly.

If you scored 2 points:
Maybe you're feeling a little stressed, or maybe you are finding it difficult to recover from a recent traumatic event. You might have a feeling that something just 'isn't quite right' – but you can't put your finger on it. Everyone has times when it can be difficult to deal with the problems life throws at us. The good news is that there are plenty of ways to get your mental fitness levels up. Just carry on reading through the book for tips and advice.

If you scored between 3 and 11:
It's probably no surprise to hear that your mind isn't as on top of things as it could be. It might be something in particular that's getting you down, or just a general cloud of anxiety hanging over you, the reason for which isn't easy to put your finger on. **Whatever the cause, now is the time to take action**.

You must always try and remember that no matter how bad you are feeling right now, you don't have to feel this way forever. In fact, the sooner you take action to try and make things better, the easier it will be to get – and stay – on top of your anxieties. You could:
- read through the rest of this book to pick up some useful tips and helpful contacts
- talk through your feelings with family or friends, or with an organisation like the Samaritans (call 08457 909090)
- make an appointment to talk to your doctor about the way you are

feeling. It's not unusual to need help dealing with our feelings – one in four of us will have problems with our mental health at some point in our lives and your GP won't find anything strange about it.

> **For a closer look at getting through your anxieties, see *Real Life Issues: Coping With Life*.**

So what makes you stressed? One factor that affects all of us is the pace of life we lead. Many of us are very busy, with more to do and less time to do it in. The following chapter outlines just how much twenty-first century life can contribute to stress.

CHAPTER TWO:

BUSY LIVES
Finding a balance

By now you should have an idea of whether what you are experiencing can be described as stress. You'll know how and why your body is reacting to certain situations, and you'll recognise the triggers or 'stressors' that are setting off your feelings of anxiety. But why do you feel the way you do?

One thing that affects us all is having such busy lives. Being busy can make us feel like we're achieving a lot every day. But running from A to B, having to juggle school activities with home life, studying, revision, and trying to fit in some fun time too, can be a tall order.

If you're feeling tired and stressed because you have too much going on, lots of after-school activities for example, you might feel better if you drop something, even if it's just for a term. Having a lot on – even if it's all fun – can make you feel stressed by keeping you busy all the time. On the other hand, if problems at home are bugging you, some (but not too many!) after-school activities may actually help you relax and feel better.

Why not try out these relaxation exercises? They'll help you start feeling a little bit calmer.

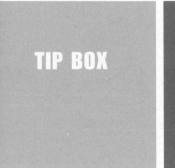

TIP BOX

Inhale (breathe in) slowly and deeply through your nose, and then exhale (breathe out) slowly through your mouth. Do this two to four times, but don't take in too much air too quickly because it can make you feel light-headed and dizzy.

And this is a good relaxation technique, especially if you're having trouble sleeping:

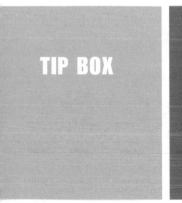

TIP BOX

Tense and relax your muscles slowly, starting at your toes and working your way up your body. Tense and relax your toes. Then do the same with your toes and your ankles. Then your toes, ankles, and calves. Then toes, ankles, calves, and thighs. Keep going up your body until you get to the top of your head!

You can do exercises like these at any time, without anyone noticing.

THE BURNOUT SCALE

There are four stages of stress. Stage 1 is a mild form of stress, the beginnings of uncertainty and worry. As you go down the list to stages 2, 3 and 4, the problem becomes more serious.

Where are you on the burnout scale?

- Stage 1 – you've begun to feel a lack of energy and enthusiasm and started to have feelings of uncertainty. You're worrying that you can't cope.
- Stage 2 – you're feeling tired and worried and think you're stagnating. You're blaming other people more and more for things going wrong and are getting more irritated. You feel like you've got too much on and worry that you're not managing your time very well.
- Stage 3 – you're generally unhappy with life. Your self-esteem is low and you're finding it hard to commit to anything. You're probably starting to feel more angry and resentful and find it hard to enjoy anything that you do.
- Stage 4 – you're beginning to withdraw from everything around you and feel like you've failed. You feel like nobody understands you. You don't talk to friends or parents as much as you should, and perhaps you're missing days from school more regularly. You might even have turned to drugs or alcohol to help you cope.

FINDING A BALANCE

Probably the best advice on how to beat stress is to make sure you have a balanced life. That means everything you do gets equal time. Make sure you keep your **SELF** in mind: **S**leep, **E**xercise, **L**eisure (something fun!) and **F**ood. If you take care of yourself by eating properly, exercising and making sure you enjoy some leisure time too, you'll probably start to feel much less stressed out.

FACT BOX

The psychiatric treatment of stress-related illnesses costs the UK £3 billion a year.

Stress can present itself in many different forms. Two in particular are panic attacks and phobias.

PANIC ATTACKS

The stress that we feel can sometimes present itself in a very physical way. Panic attacks are a good example of this. They are very common: one person in ten suffers from panic attacks.

A panic attack is defined as a quick onset of intense fear or discomfort, which peaks after approximately 10 minutes, and includes at least four of the following symptoms:

- a feeling of imminent danger or doom
- the need to escape
- palpitations
- sweating
- trembling
- shortness of breath or feeling of being smothered
- a feeling of choking
- chest pain or discomfort
- nausea or abdominal discomfort
- dizziness or light headedness
- a sense of things being unreal, depersonalisation
- a fear of losing control or 'going crazy'
- a fear of dying
- tingling sensations
- chills or hot flushes.

You might suffer a panic attack out of the blue or you might always get them in certain situations, for example every time you enter a tunnel.

How often you get them and how bad they feel varies from person to person. One person might suffer repeated attacks for weeks, while someone else will have short bouts of very severe attacks.

Many people who suffer from panic attacks become convinced that the attacks indicate something more seriously wrong with their bodies, maybe an undiagnosed illness. Others arrange a fixed daily routine to try to avoid the possibility of getting an attack. For those people, it makes it impossible to go outside their safety zone without suffering severe anxiety.

Most people who suffer from panic disorders do so between late adolescence and their mid-thirties.

PHOBIAS

Phobias are really common, so if you have one you're by no means alone. In fact, it's estimated that one person in ten experiences this type of intense anxiety.

Phobias are emotional and physical reactions to feared objects or situations. Symptoms can include:
- feelings of panic, dread, horror, or terror
- rapid heartbeat, shortness of breath, trembling, and an overwhelming desire to run away – all the physical reactions associated with extreme fear.

It's possible to develop a fear of almost anything and there are hundreds of officially recognised phobias, from arachnophobia (the fear of spiders) to zoophobia (the fear of animals generally). Some are quite unusual. Did you know that if you are lachanophobic you have a fear of vegetables? Or that alektorophobia is a fear of chickens?

Whatever the phobia, the sufferer will experience stress and anxiety when they're faced with the object of their fear.

Some phobias are easier to manage than others, and affect people at particular times or in specific places. If you're scared of heights, you can usually avoid tall buildings or looking over the edge of cliffs. If you're scared of the dark, you might try going to sleep with a light on.

These steps don't take away the phobia, but they will help you not to encounter your fear. But if you find your phobia affects the way you want to live your everyday life, you may find it completely takes over your life.

There are lots of theories about the best way to help you overcome your phobia. Here are some suggestions:

- Try some relaxation techniques like yoga or meditation to calm you down and help deal with the anxiety
- At a time when you don't feel stressed or threatened, make a list of exactly what you feel when your phobia is triggered
- Breaking down your phobia into stages of anxiety can really help. By listing how it affects you mentally and physically, and what you think would happen in your very worst-case scenario, you will be able to anticipate what you will feel before it happens
- Physical exercise can also help. By exercising the heart, you'll be making it stronger and less likely to trigger the rapid heartbeat that makes anxiety feel so unpleasant
- Hypnotism can sometimes help with phobias. Hypnosis involves trying to look beyond your conscious thoughts by exploring your subconscious mind. But always check with your GP to see if they think it would work for you.

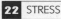

EXERCISE THAT STRESS AWAY

How you look after yourself is crucial in dealing with a major symptom of your busy life: stress.

Stress can in some cases raise your blood pressure and lead to heart disease. But a good way of keeping those symptoms at bay is by taking cardiovascular exercise. That's the kind of exercise that works on your heart and lungs and gets your blood pumping around your body more efficiently. It includes activities like swimming, power walking, cycling, jogging and aerobics. These activities all release **endorphins**, your body's natural painkillers.

Endorphins also reduce stress, depression and anxiety. So taking up aerobics, for example, is a great way to bust that stress. Exercise is also a good outlet for all those negative emotions you feel when you're stressed. Regular exercise can improve your mood and you might just find yourself with a more positive outlook on life.

The ways you react to stressful situations can be as different as the many reasons you get stressed. In the next chapter we'll look at some of the most common triggers for stress. Exams, relationships and bullying are just a few examples. Alongside them are some useful remedies for coping.

CHAPTER THREE:

THINGS THAT STRESS YOU OUT
A few things that lead to stress

Being busy is just one factor that can lead to feelings of anxiety or not being able to cope. There are of course lots of different **stressors** that affect us to varying degrees. What bothers you might not affect someone else half as much. But here are some common stressors that affect many teenagers.

EXAMS

The run-up to exams can be especially worrying. You might need to get certain grades, and feel that if you don't, you'll be letting everyone – including yourself – down.

Think about how you are feeling:
- out of control?
- panicked?
- are you having trouble sleeping?
- are you eating more/less than usual?

These are all signs that your looming exams are causing you stress.

If you're stressed by exams, you're by no means alone. The number of young people calling the free helpline ChildLine because they are struggling to cope with the pressure of exams rose by 50 per cent last year.

'Some children who call ChildLine tell us that exams are the "last straw" in their young lives – they may be suffering abuse, their families may be going through a break-up or they may be being bullied. Tragically a small number of children who call ChildLine have harmed themselves or have even attempted to commit suicide because they are struggling to cope with the pressure of exams.' **Carole Easton, Chief Executive, ChildLine**

Try to remember that, while exams are important, if you don't get the grade you want, you've still got plenty of options. You'd be surprised at how many people have got to the top without having a load of A-grade certificates. Did you know that both Albert Einstein and Richard Branson did badly at school? Einstein is regarded as a genius and Branson, who created the Virgin brand, is one of the richest men in the world.

There are people who can help you get through this stressful period by giving you some good advice about how best to prepare for your exams. Your teacher's a great starting point, although some teachers

are more approachable than others, and you might find they're
hassling you more than helping you! If that's the case, why not try
talking to your friends about how they organise their revision?

You could always try some of these tips, too:
- The odd hour of revision here and there isn't enough. Make a
  revision plan you can stick to, with a daily outline that includes
  times for breaks and meals
- Know what your good and worst subjects are and then mix them
  up on your timetable – don't do all the nightmare topics at once
- Set targets that you know you can reach and tick them off as you
  accomplish them
- Get help from teachers or parents, friends or websites
- Find somewhere quiet to revise. You could also try working with
  other people, but if you can't concentrate, save get-togethers for
  breaks from the books
- Put your exams into perspective – they're just one aspect of life.

Having to get certain grades can make you feel scared. Whether it's
the expectation from your mum, dad or carer, or whether the
expectation comes from you yourself, the pressure is immense.

You might find yourself experiencing some of the typical symptoms of
stress – mood changes, poor appetite, lack of sleep, and even suicidal
thoughts, for example. But stress can also affect motivation, making it
even harder to study for exams.

These tips are a good way of starting to control your situation and
feelings, rather than letting them get the better of you.

Manage your studying

Don't go mad and lock yourself in with your books 24 hours a day.
Two to three hours is the maximum amount of time you can study
before you stop really taking in what you read. So remember to give
yourself regular breaks. And a few treats now and again will do
wonders for your motivation!

Get enough sleep

Exam stress sometimes makes it difficult to get a good night's sleep.
So set a definite time to go to bed and stick to it. Relaxing before you
go to bed, by having a bubble bath, reading or listening to music, can
help you sleep.

Keep busy

Keeping busy when you're not studying will help stop you worrying
about your exams. Try a sport, take up painting or do anything you
enjoy.

Be nice to yourself

Self-affirmation works wonders! You may feel silly but tell yourself that
you are great, you can do it, and generally psych yourself up to a
feeling that you will come top. Why do you think sportsmen and
women do this before a match?

Exam time can cause a huge amount of stress. But by getting a good

*Remember – if you want something
in your life to change you have to do
something different.*

study routine in place and following some relaxation tips as well, you can begin to take control of your feelings and anxieties.

FAMILY LIFE

School life may be a major source of pressure, but it's unlikely to be the only one. Family life can also present its own problems. As the saying goes, 'You can choose your friends but you can't choose your family.' It might sometimes feel like you're living in a soap opera with the amount of drama that goes on at home. You might be dealing with divorce or money problems and you might feel that nobody at home really understands you.

Recent research carried out in Sweden found that more and more children are suffering from persistent headaches. The teenagers interviewed blamed schoolwork, but in fact it was the worry caused by family life that led to tension and headaches. In Britain, one in five teenagers suffer from headaches.

Headaches are just one symptom of stress caused by family life. There may be a whole host of other things you've noticed about yourself that can be related to your anxieties: feeling more withdrawn, suffering mood swings or just not getting enough sleep are all signs of stress.

Parents

As you get into your teenage years, your relationship with your mum, dad or carer will be tested to the full. It will certainly be a period of anxiety for you.

- Are you doing your homework?
- Why do you spend so much time on the telephone? It costs money, you know!
- Are you sure that boy/girl is right for you?

- Why did you come in so late last night?
- So what are you going to do with your future?

Sounds familiar? The people who look after you – your parents or carers – are still a pretty big part of your life, but you might feel trapped by the way they treat you. You might think they're still treating you like a kid, even though you're growing up; and that's bound to annoy you and make you feel that they are worrying about you for nothing.

Sometimes you're going to argue with them, rebel against them, even ignore them.

There are 7.5 million teenagers living in the UK. A recent survey published on the BBC News website found that a third of teenagers don't feel loved or cared for by their parents. That means two and a half million young people feel alone.

Arguing

Whether it's full-blown fights or constant sniping, not getting on with your brother, sister or any other member of your family can be a real pain. You may not always be best friends, but you can learn to respect each other.

Try the following ideas: they might just make things a bit more bearable.

- Think about why you fight so much – is it about being the best? Or are you too stubborn to give in? Maybe you're using each other as emotional punch bags because you're stressed about something else?
- When you're both feeling calm, try to start a discussion about why

you fight so much. Work out what triggers the fights and how you can avoid them
■ Don't be afraid to let your family member know the rows are bothering you – they won't want to cause so much stress
■ Try to take a deep breath instead of just lashing out.

You might feel like you're the only one with family problems. Don't worry, because arguments at home are much more common than you think: arguing is normal.

Real arguments, the ones where both sides feel absolutely passionate about an issue – are an ordinary and healthy part of family life. Ordinary because any family who says they don't argue is either lying or secretly living with years of pent up frustration. Healthy because repressing strong emotions and opinions isn't good for your head! Talking about a problem when it comes up might cause an argument, but it might not – so why not take a chance?

GET WHAT YOU WANT ... THE RIGHT WAY

There is an art to getting what you want that doesn't involve slamming the door! The first thing to do is to say what you want and why. Be clear and calm. Then listen to the other side of the argument, without interrupting. Try to understand their point of view and, most important, don't be too rigid in what you want. Compromise – that means reaching a conclusion that each side is happy with. You never know, it might set the tone for future debates!

Sibling rivalry

The majority of families have two children in them, which means you are more than likely have a sister or brother to put up with – and that can lead to feelings of envy, frustration and a lifetime of sibling rivalry.

Did you know that sibling rivalry is a basic animal instinct? A litter of newborn puppies will tussle for the best space, the first feed and the most affection from the mother. When you think about it, fighting with your brother or sister isn't so different. Don't most of your arguments come down to fighting for your own space, fighting for attention or fighting out of jealousy? There's nothing wrong with a bit of healthy competition.

That said, sibling rivalry plays a big part in teenage stress. So how do you deal with it?

- Being competitive can be a motivating force, but don't let it get out of hand. If you find yourself getting aggressive over the slightest thing, it's time to take a deep breath
- Sibling rivalry is a habit you can break. Let your brother or sister know how you feel now and start working at it. You might be able to salvage a perfectly good, even strong, relationship
- If you resent your sibling because you feel they get more support and attention from your parents than you do, they're not to blame! Tell your parents how you feel; you've got nothing to lose
- Stop jealousy in its tracks by remembering that there is enough love to go around. Focus on all the positive things you have in your life, too.

ANA'S STORY

'My parents were separated and I lived with my mum and younger brother, Adam. He always seemed to get attention and my mum always did what he wanted to do. I'd always ask if we could catch a movie or go shopping for some new gear but she'd always make an excuse involving Adam. In the end I couldn't stand it. I moved out and lived with my dad for a week. I think I made the point and when I

returned home to my mum's things weren't perfect, but I think she understood that I needed some quality time and attention too.'

Ana's story isn't unusual. Sibling rivalry, arguments and tension between brothers and sisters can cause a whole load of upset and stress. Remember, everyone with a kid brother or sister feels the same at some point or other.

Why not try this exercise to help you calm down? It only takes five minutes – or longer if you want it to. Make sure you're feeling safe and comfortable.

TIP BOX

Imagine yourself in a walled garden at the time of the year you like the most.

As you wander around you notice an old-fashioned door in one of the walls. You make your way over and open the door. On the other side is your very own safe space, anywhere you want, with or without people. This is your special place where no one can get to you. Enjoy being there and when you're ready make your way back to the door, closing it firmly. Then walk around the garden again and open your eyes when you are ready. Remember, this place is there for you any time you need it.

BULLYING

Exams and family life affect everyone's stress levels at some point in their lives. But another major factor of stress is bullying, and that can feel a bit more difficult to deal with.

Nearly everyone is bullied at some time in their lives: by brothers and sisters, by neighbours, by adults or by other children. If you are being bullied, you're bound to feel scared, vulnerable and quite alone.

Did you know that these people were bullied when they were younger?
- Tom Cruise
- Ms Dynamite
- Gareth Gates
- David Beckham
- Sarah Cox.

They're all really successful people now, though. For some, the bullying went on for years; for others it was less frequent. Bullying is wrong and it's never your fault. **Remember – no one deserves to be bullied**.

Think about how the bullying makes you feel. Anxious and stressed? Do you worry about your situation at night, can't sleep, skip school and generally feel alone?

More than two-thirds of teenagers in England wouldn't find it easy to tell a teacher if they were being bullied – because they believe they would not be taken seriously or would suffer reprisals as a result of 'telling'.

ChildLine, 2003

It may not always be easy to tell someone you're being bullied, but the following tips might help you start feeling more in control of the situation:

- Tell a friend what is happening. Ask him or her to help you. It will be harder for the bully to pick on you if you have a friend with you for support.
- Try to ignore the bullying or say 'No' really firmly, then turn and walk away. Don't worry if people think you are running away. Remember, it's very hard for the bully to go on bullying someone who won't stand still to listen.
- Try not to show that you are upset or angry. Bullies love to get a reaction – it's 'fun'. If you can keep calm and hide your emotions, they might get bored and leave you alone. As one teenager said to us, 'they can't bully you if you don't care'.
- Don't fight back if you can help it. Most bullies are bigger or stronger than you. If you fight back you could make the situation worse, get hurt or be blamed for starting the trouble.
- It's not worth getting hurt to keep possessions or money. If you feel threatened, give the bullies what they want. Property can be replaced; you can't.
- Try to think up funny or clever replies in advance. Make a joke of it. Replies don't have to be wonderfully brilliant or clever but it helps to have an answer ready. Practise saying them in the mirror at home. Using prepared replies works best if the bully is not too threatening and just needs to be put off. The bully might just decide that you are too clever to pick on.
- Try to avoid being alone in the places where you know the bully is likely to pick on you. This might mean changing your route to school, avoiding parts of the playground, or only using common rooms or lavatories when other people are there. It's not fair that you have to do this, but it might put the bully off.

■ Sometimes asking the bully to repeat what they said can put them off. Often bullies are not brave enough to repeat the remark exactly so they tone it down. If they repeat it, you will have made them do something they hadn't planned on and this gives you some control of the situation.

■ Keep a diary of what is happening. Write down details of the incidents and your feelings. When you do decide to tell someone, a written record of the bullying makes it easier to prove what has been going on.

> **For a closer look at bullying, see**
> ***Real Life Issues: Bullying.***

There are plenty of stressful events in your life, like bullying, that you can take control of, given the right advice and support. But there are some others you can do nothing about. Puberty is one example and the next chapter will help you understand the changes affecting your body.

TIP BOX

Remember – you can if you think you can.

CHAPTER FOUR:

GROWING PAINS
Your changing body

As you go through your teenage years, your body experiences a whole range of changes. You might also be starting to become more self-conscious and shy. How you look becomes more important than ever and having enough confidence to cope with the physical changes that are happening can affect the way you feel and deal with life.

Everything about you is starting to change: the way you look, the way you feel about yourself, emotions and friendships. No wonder you're suffering from anxiety overload!

The changes that happen during your early teenage years, although they affect so much of your body and mind, are best described by one word: **puberty**.

Puberty is the name for the time when your body begins to develop and change as you move from child to adult. Among other things, for girls this means developing breasts, and for boys it means starting to look more like a man. During puberty, your body will grow faster than at any other time in your life, except for when you were a baby.

Understanding the changes that puberty causes before they happen can help deal with the stress that also comes with puberty.

TIME TO CHANGE

Puberty usually starts between the ages of eight and 13 in girls and between ten and 15 in boys. Some people begin a bit earlier or later than that, and you can experience puberty-related changes at any point during those years. That may help explain why some of your friends still look like young kids while others look more like adults.

One of the first signs of puberty is hair growing where it didn't grow before. Boys and girls both begin to grow hair under their arms and in their pubic areas (on and around the genitals).

When your body is ready to begin puberty, your pituitary gland (a pea-shaped gland located at the bottom of your brain) releases special hormones. Depending on whether you're a boy or a girl, these hormones go to work on different parts of the body. For boys, that means the production of sperm. And for girls, it means preparing your body for periods and future pregnancy.

TAKING SHAPE

Your body also fills out and changes shape during puberty. A boy's shoulders will grow wider, and his body will become more muscular. You might notice a bit of breast growth on your chest. Don't worry, this is normal – and for most boys it goes away by the end of puberty. In addition, boys' voices crack and eventually become deeper, their penises grow longer and wider, their testes get bigger.

If you're a girl, you might notice your body becoming more curvy. You'll gain weight on your hips, and notice your breasts developing.

Is your body shaping up in the way you want or expect it to? Puberty is stressful. How your body shapes up as an adult has a huge impact on how you feel about yourself. Whether you have the right breast size or a decent six-pack can affect your sense of worth. And what if you're an early or a late developer?

Do you worry about looking different from your friends and other people in your year? Being taller or flat-chested; still having a high-pitched voice; or feeling stressed because your body seems all out of proportion? Changes take time and there's not a lot you can do just yet about changing the way you look, but you can have more faith in yourself.

> **For a closer look at confidence levels, look at**
> ***Real Life Issues: Confidence and Self-Esteem.***

With all this growing and developing going on, girls will notice an increase in their body fat – that's quite normal. Gaining some weight is part of becoming a woman.

But getting stressed about how much you eat and becoming too concerned with your body image can put both your physical and mental health at risk. The Eating Disorders Association estimates that around 165,000 people in the UK are currently being treated for eating disorders, with many more remaining undiagnosed. Anyone can develop an eating disorder. Women aged between 15 and 25 are the most likely to do so, but this problem doesn't affect only females. A growing number of young men are now also suffering.

> **For a closer look at eating disorders, see**
> ***Real Life issues: Eating Disorders.***

ROLLERCOASTER EMOTIONS

Just as those hormones change the way your body looks on the outside, they also create changes on the inside. During puberty, you might feel confused or experience strong emotions that you've never had before. You might feel over-sensitive or become upset easily, find yourself getting irritable with friends and family and most likely feel anxious about your changing body.

Sometimes it can be hard to deal with the stress that all these new emotions bring with them. It's important to know that while your body is adjusting to the new hormones, so is your mind. Try to remember that people usually aren't trying to hurt your feelings or upset you on purpose. It might not be your family or friends – it might be your new 'puberty brain' trying to adjust.

DEVELOPING DIFFERENTLY

People are all a little different from each other, so it makes sense that they don't all develop in the same way. During puberty, everyone changes at his or her own pace. Maybe some of your friends are getting curves, and you don't have any yet. Maybe your best friend's voice has changed, and you think you still sound like a kid. Or maybe you're sick of being the tallest girl in your class or the only boy who has to shave.

But just about everyone catches up eventually, and most differences between you and your friends will even out. Until then, hang in there. Puberty can be quite a wild ride! Remember that models such as Kate Moss and movie stars such as Julia Roberts were known at school for being too tall/too thin/having goofy teeth, and look at them now!

As you get older, you might find yourself in a love–hate relationship with your body. The next chapter outlines some of the reasons we get so anxious about the way we look and tells you how you can overcome any stressful feelings you may have about your appearance.

CHAPTER FIVE:

I DON'T LIKE MY BODY!
Unrealistic expectations

Most people have hang-ups about their body – or bits of it – at some point in their lives, but did you know ...?

- Girls get it worse. Researchers at Glasgow University found that women are up to ten times more likely to feel unhappy with their body image than men – often seeing themselves as overweight even when they're a healthy weight for their height.

- The number of men suffering from body dysmorphic disorder (extreme dissatisfaction with the body) is rising. Men tend to be more concerned with their skin (especially acne and scarring), hair loss, nose and genital size, and not feeling muscular enough.

- Research in Canada and the UK suggests that the wealthier you are, the more likely you are to dislike your body. Experts think there's more pressure on the wealthy to achieve the thin 'ideal' because they have the money to do so and are more exposed to media imagery. Europe has much higher levels of body image dissatisfaction than less developed countries.

The way you feel about your body can lead to a lot of anxiety, with negative and confidence-crushing feelings taking over, especially after puberty's done its job.

Experts think that the media plays a part – with all those images of skinny women and muscly men – but that the major causes are much more complicated and more likely to be about our own, deep-rooted feelings of self-worth.

People who overcome these illnesses often describe eating as the only thing they could control in a time when they felt unable to cope with other events or emotions. These are just some of the triggers:

- Setting high standards for yourself, or feeling pressured by others
- Feeling anxious about the natural weight gain that happens during puberty, or fearing adulthood and the responsibilities it brings
- Suffering low self-esteem, possibly due to bullying
- Stress caused by problems with your family, friends, partner, job or study
- Traumatic events like death or divorce

TIP BOX

Recognising that you have a problem is the first step to getting better.

So how can you begin to celebrate your body? Let's start with a reality check.

MEDIA HYPE

Every day you're exposed to hundreds of media images through television, films, magazines, newspapers, websites and advertising. All these feature beautiful people selling beautiful dreams. But are they really that beautiful?

Cover shots today use flattering lighting, enhanced make-up and airbrushing – an art that's used on loads of magazine pictures and posters.

'Airbrushing means that we can do almost anything to a model's face – to the point that we can book a model who isn't quite right because we know we can change the bits we don't like later. For example, we can thin or thicken lips, whiten and straighten teeth, zap wrinkles, shadows and blemishes, change make-up and skin colour, adjust hairstyles and even trim off any unwanted bulges.'

Claire, Art Director on a glossy magazine

Let's face it, looking good is the job of a model or a celebrity. Most of them will have access to personal trainers, hairdressers, make-up artists, stylists and even personal chefs. If you had all of this, wouldn't you look gorgeous too?

Despite looking great, however, being a celebrity is a competitive industry and lots of stars have insecurities.

But it's not just girls who feel stressed about the way they look. Boys and men, too, are increasingly feeling the pressure of looking good. Eating disorders and body image problems are conditions affecting more and more males today.

FACT BOX

According to the British Medical Association, many models and actresses have only 10–15 per cent body fat (the healthy range is 22–26 per cent), making them not only underweight, but also at risk of ill health.

The fact is, however great today's celebrities look, many of them are exercising too much, eating too little or getting cosmetic surgery in order to achieve the perfect body image. And don't beat yourself up too much about not having that perfect six-pack – that rippling torso you saw in *Snatch* didn't belong to Brad Pitt. He has a body double!

TAKE ACTION

Think about some important points:

- Don't believe everything you see. The pictures you see in magazines aren't always what they seem, and many images can be constructed, manipulated, unreal. Let's face it, even celebrities look bad first thing in the morning.
- Stop comparing yourself with media images and start concentrating on doing what you can do with what you have. Exercise regularly, eat healthily and remember to relax!
- Working out until you feel faint or starving yourself to get rid of body fat isn't clever, it's unhealthy. Pale, drawn and lethargic, or rosy-cheeked and energetic – which do you prefer?

Try to stay in touch with reality. When you feel bombarded by media beauties, take a look around you. We come in all sorts of shapes and sizes. There's no right or wrong way to look.

Feeling great about yourself can give you confidence, especially when it comes to relationships. They will without a doubt provide you with many sleepless nights and the following chapter looks more closely at some of the stressful situations that finding love can put you in.

CHAPTER SIX:

RELATIONSHIPS
You're a whole, not a half

As your body changes, so does the way you feel. You've probably noticed that you're more self-conscious these days, more anxious about how you look and what you wear. What other people think of you matters a lot more than it used to.

And sometimes, what certain people think – especially people you fancy – can become a major concern.

Normally, a fair amount of anxiety and stress goes hand-in-hand with finding love, and even just thinking about how to get your perfect partner can cause the butterflies in your stomach to go wild.

If you're not going out with anyone, you might feel even more anxious about relationships. You might find yourself worrying about the reasons you don't have a girlfriend or boyfriend, and before you know it, your self-esteem can reach an all-time low.

Have you ever thought any of the following?
■ I'm too ugly to get a boyfriend or girlfriend

- I'm too fat/thin
- I'm too spotty
- I'm too boring
- I don't like the right music
- I don't wear the right clothes
- I don't know how to kiss properly.

When you get these thoughts, pamper yourself – get a new haircut or some new clothes, buy a CD or rent a movie – anything that makes you feel good again. It might just give you the boost you need to start dealing with your own self-confidence. And also check out *Real Life Issues: Confidence and Self Esteem*.

All relationships mean compromise. When you're single you only have to worry about yourself. Your time is your own, so make the most of it. Have some fun and grab everything that life has to offer.

You won't meet anyone new if you always hang around in the same crowd. Increase your circle of friends. Take up a sport or another activity. Put yourself in a situation where you're likely to meet the kind of person you'd like as a potential partner.

Looking after number one is important: confidence is the most attractive attribute you can have. Appearing desperate is a real turn-off. Enjoy life to the full, whether you're single or in a couple. A relationship will come along but, until it does, single life can be a lot of fun.

Of course, dealing with relationships is hard enough. But teenage years also bring with them uncertain feelings and anxieties about sexuality.

EXPLORING YOUR SEXUALITY

No one is born knowing who they are, let alone whether they're gay, straight or whatever. Some people are predominately attracted to people of the same sex. They're gay or lesbian. Others are attracted to both men and women to varying degrees. They're bisexual. You can change, so take your time. It's OK to be unsure.

Deciding on your sexuality can be a confusing and stressful time. There's a pressure to conform and if you don't, it's easy for anxieties to overwhelm you.

At some point in your life, you're bound to feel attracted to someone of the same sex. But that doesn't necessarily mean you're gay. For many people, these feelings are just part of normal sexual development and many go on to have relationships with people of the opposite sex.

What if these feelings don't go away but get stronger?

- If you're asking questions about your sexuality, then you're probably not ready to give yourself a label. Working it out takes time.
- Nobody knows what makes someone gay, lesbian, bisexual or straight. You don't choose your sexuality. It's not due to your upbringing or the people you hang around with. Sometimes it just 'is'.
- Being gay, lesbian or bisexual is normal. You haven't done anything wrong. Unfortunately, not everyone sees it that way. Some people feel threatened by things they don't understand. Because of this, you may be tempted to keep quiet or pretend that you're heterosexual. The trouble is, you can't hide your feelings forever.

What's more, you shouldn't have to. You have a right to be proud of who you are.

■ It can feel isolating to discover that your sexuality is different from that of your friends, particularly if you don't know anyone else who's gay or lesbian. It's good to talk to like-minded people. There are plenty of national and local support groups.

> **For a closer look at these issues, see**
> **_Real Life Issues: Sex and Relationships._**

SPLITTING UP

Everyone has relationship problems at one point or other in their lives – probably several, in all honesty! But nothing ever prepares you for how you're going to feel when things start to go pear-shaped.

You might feel angry and confused, especially if you want things to go back to the way they were. And even if it was you who ended a relationship, you might not really be sure about why you decided to do it. Talking about how you feel can help lift your feelings of despair.

Splitting up is a confusing time. Emotions aren't always black and white and you can spend days and weeks feeling anxious about what you should do. Not all relationships are meant to be. And in the long run, it's much better to admit when something is finished rather than letting it drag on. Knowing that you dealt with it decently will mean you can leave the relationship with your head held high.

Getting over someone

Unfortunately there is no magic trick to help you move on.

The first few days and weeks are going to be the worst. Staying in and

being miserable is a part of the healing process, but try to avoid
dragging it out too much. Don't let your negative feelings take over,
and try not to spend day after day worrying about what you did wrong.

If they don't want to be with you any more, that's up to them – it's
their loss at the end of the day.

You're a whole, not a half

The first time you experience stress as a singleton you may feel extra
uncomfortable. If your partner used to listen to your problems or talk
things through with you, you'll need to find a new support network.
Remember your friends and family? They were there before your
partner and they're probably still there now. Renew the ties. They'll
understand and will help you through difficulties.

Resist the temptation to ring up your ex and chat like you used to: this
prevents you moving on. You need to find other people to help you.

Relationships break down for a variety of reasons. Try not to get too
worked up or sad about it. It wasn't all your fault and you aren't a
failure because it didn't work out. Learn from the experience and it will
help you recognise the right person when they come along.

> **For a closer look at dealing with relationships,
> see *Real Life Issues: Sex and Relationships*.**

Relationships will continue to be a source of worry and anxiety well
into your adult life. But learning how to manage your feelings can help
you cope. And thinking about your future doesn't just involve who your
partner in life will be – there are many other issues about your future
that are bound to be on your mind.

CHAPTER SEVEN:

WHERE'S THE FUTURE?
Career choices, money matters

By the time you've reached sixteen, you're probably not feeling much like a child any more. Or maybe the thought of becoming an adult, and taking on everything that involves, scares you.

Emotionally, this is a really hard time for you, because things aren't as straightforward as they used to be.

The biggest questions for 16–18-year-olds are:
- where am I going?
- what am I going to do to get there?
- how am I going to make money?

These aren't easy questions, and lots of people – even those in their 20s and 30s – say 'I don't know what I'm going to do ...' So remember, it's perfectly normal to be uncertain about the future, whatever your age.

You might not feel that you have any dreams or abilities, but you'd be surprised. The best thing to do is to keep thinking about it. Make a list

of the things (both inside school and out) that you:
- enjoy
- think you're good at
- know other people think you're good at.

Try and put them in order – write down those that are most important. It might also help to talk to friends about your hopes and worries for the future. They'll probably have the same sorts of feelings as you. And you can always try talking to your parents or other adults and see what advice they give you – remember, it's up to you whether or not you take their advice.

And why not get in touch with a Connexions personal adviser, through your school or college or local youth centre? A Connexions personal adviser's job is to support you and provide you with information about courses and work opportunities, and he or she can help link you up with other organisations, too.

Take your time. Don't panic, just because you don't know what you want to do just yet.

MONEY MATTERS

Thinking about your future may be weighing heavily on your mind. There are decisions to make about careers, jobs, apprenticeships, courses, etc. It's not easy to be certain about which you should go for. Thinking that you have to get it right can make you feel worried and confused.

Also, as independence looms, you'll be wondering exactly how to balance all your oncoming responsibilities. Money, for example can be the cause of much worry and although you don't have to manage your own finances just yet, the future can provide you with anxious thoughts.

'I'm wondering how I will manage my money. How will I balance it all and learn to deal with it? It used to be so simple.'

Alex

One financial term you probably hear a lot about already is debt. Worrying about taking out loans and getting into difficulty with your money can be an issue for you even before you become financially independent.

Debt

Lots of people experience difficulty with finances. It can be especially hard when you first become independent and have to begin paying for rent and bills.

It doesn't matter how much money you have coming in – it's very unusual to find someone who hasn't spent more than they've earned at some point in their life.

FACT BOX

State of the nation
As a country we owe nearly a trillion pounds of personal debt.

Deciding whether or not to go to college can bring all sorts of different worries and emotions. You're likely to be anxious about which is the right course for you. One deciding factor we hear a lot about in the news is the cost of further education. Student poverty is well highlighted in the media and taking out a student loan can add to the pressure of deciding what to do next. Ending your academic life in debt is a reality for many young people, but you can find a way through it.

If you find you are getting into debt:
- Try keeping a list of everything you spend to find out where the money goes
- Prioritise your spending. For example, put aside money for things like rent, bills (if you're not living at home or in a hall of residence) and food first, then clothes, entertainment and luxuries after that
- Set yourself a budget and stick to it. But remember, treats are allowed from time to time!
- Think about ways of increasing your income, such as taking on a bar job or working in a shop at weekends.

Calculating how much money you have coming in and what you have going out is vital to staying on top of your finances.

You should also take a look at *Real Life Issues: Money*, which gives you a lowdown on all the financial jargon – the meaning of debit, credit, interest, current account, savings account, Chip and PIN, overdraft, etc. It'll also give you information about exactly what's in your wallet – what a debit card is, how it works, and the ins and outs of credit and store charge cards too.

Benefits

As a rule, students aren't eligible for benefits, and some benefits aren't available to people under 18. But if you're feeling desperate to stand on your own two feet and want to move out of home then it's worth looking into benefits.

There are all types of pressures on you right now, whether they're knocking on your door or likely to be an issue in a couple of years' time. It's likely you'll have thought of and most probably worried about financial matters. One area to consider and certainly look into is claiming for benefits.

It might be difficult to get the benefits or income you need to be independent. The benefits system is complicated and the rules change a lot. So it's useful to speak to someone who knows the system. You could:

■ ask your friends and family to help you fill in difficult forms
■ look in your local phone book for your nearest Citizens Advice Bureau – they can help you look into what you're entitled to and also help with filling out forms.

As you think about your looming independence, fleeing the nest is bound to cause stress. It might not be on the cards just yet, but in a few years' time, leaving home will be a potentially stressful reality.

MOVING OUT

Looking for a new place to live might not be a priority for you just now, but becoming more independent probably is. And in a couple of years' time, moving out could well be an issue that brings along worry and frustration.

If you are an older teenager, you might be on the point of leaving for college or you may have decided to move out and find a job. But where do you begin? The comforts that home life can bring are going to be pretty tough to beat, and deciding on what you move into can present all kinds of stress.

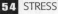

One option that's open to you is renting, but be prepared. A good pair of shoes and a notepad and pen are essential!

Flats for rent are generally advertised in local papers, estate agents, college notice boards, post office windows and online. You can even find out information about the area you are considering moving to online.

What's the maximum you can afford? Don't be tempted to go for something beyond your price range. Decide on your limits and stick to them. Then make a list of what your flat absolutely **must** have – central heating, a phone, close to the station, for example – and what in an ideal world you'd **like** it to have.

Decide what questions you need to ask, then make that call. Don't delay – if the flat looks like good value, you won't be the only one to have spotted it!

When you go to see it, check out the neighbourhood and make sure you'd feel comfortable walking around there, especially late at night. Once you're in the flat look carefully at its condition – if there's a problem, ask the landlord what he's going to do about it. Can you meet your future flatmates before you sign the contract?

Don't despair if you are spending hours or days on this and not finding what you want. It can take time just to work out what is good value and what you can get for your money in different areas. You don't want to start moving again six months from now, so don't settle for something second-rate unless you're really pushed for time.

Think about not just what you want, but what you can afford.

Renting a flat from a private landlord isn't the only option you've got when it comes to looking for a new place to live. You could always look at renting from your local council or trying a housing association, which might provide you with cheaper alternatives.

Contact your local council's housing department. You can get the number from your local phone book. Look in your local phone book, too, for details of housing associations in your area.

Housing may not be your number one priority right now, but whether it's in your late teens or early twenties, you're likely to be affected by the choice of where you live. And the tips given might just demystify the whole process for you, making finding a new home less of a stressful prospect.

There are plenty of things to worry about in your teenage years. We've looked at exam stress, anxieties surrounding home life and relationships, what to do if you're being bullied and also financial concerns. The feelings you have, whether high or low, will come and go.

Problems occur, though, when the lows begin to outnumber the highs. And the next chapter looks at what happens when your stress turns into depression.

CHAPTER EIGHT:

DEPRESSION
When stress turns into depression

There's a heap of challenges facing you right now, from relationships to thinking about what you do with your life.

Everything seems to be changing, and the roller-coaster emotions you're probably experiencing can be quite difficult to deal with. With so much going on right now, it's perfectly normal to feel stressed, anxious or even lonely from time to time. But for most people, these feelings will come and go.

How many of the following have you experienced?
- Being bullied at school or somewhere else
- Having trouble with your girlfriend or boyfriend, or a close friend
- Leaving home
- Someone close to you being ill or dying
- Arguments with friends or family
- Worrying about your sexuality
- Thinking about exams
- Deciding on your future
- Not liking your body.

Worrying about exams and having someone close to you die are obviously two very different experiences. But what they have in common is that both can lead to depression. It's not so much the seriousness of what happens to us as our inability to cope with the stress they bring with them that leads us to become depressed.

These days, depression amongst teenagers is regarded as a very serious problem: five out of every 100 teenagers are affected by depression.

When the stresses in your life start making you feel overwhelmed and out of control, depression usually follows. You start to lack energy, and lose the desire to get out and do things. It can also feel hard to connect with the world outside. These depressive feelings can sometimes lead to other psychological problems, including eating disorders such as anorexia and bulimia.

Sometimes it can get so bad that you feel life's not worth living any more.

FACT BOX

The Samaritans found that one in seven people between the ages of 16 and 34 have felt suicidal at some point due to stress.

HOW DO YOU KNOW IF YOU'RE DEPRESSED?

'I couldn't concentrate on my work. I was always daydreaming and wanted to sleep a lot. I couldn't be bothered to do anything.

Sometimes when I felt really low it was scary, and I'd start messing about at school, getting into trouble.'

Natalie

Do you:
- lie or make up stories?
- cry a lot?
- feel lazy or bored and tired a lot?
- steal things or get into trouble?
- have trouble sleeping or have a lot of bad dreams?
- feel you're being moody or snappy?
- eat a lot more or a lot less than usual?
- worry about things?
- feel life is not worth living?
- not want to go out?
- feel that nobody likes you or that people are talking behind your back?

If you've answered 'yes' to some or many of these questions, then it's time to get help.

'After I felt depressed a few times I knew I'd always come out of it, and just tried to do things to distract myself till it passed. That helped a bit. It was horrible thinking it might come back, though. In the end I went for counselling, which helped me feel more in control of my life.'

Tom

It's important to remember that most things can be put right if you start making the right moves to control your stress levels.

It's OK not to feel happy or positive all the time. It's always good to talk to someone about how you feel. When you do that, you start to understand why you feel a certain way and begin to feel more in control. It can be hard to talk to family and sometimes even friends, but there are many organisations that can help.

'I didn't think I could talk to anyone I knew. I thought it would just make things worse. I couldn't talk to my friends about it because I didn't think they would take it seriously. I just felt completely alone. I wrote to a problem page and they encouraged me to phone a helpline. Once I did that they helped me have more confidence to get help.'

Neil

It's important to get help so that you can start to feel that you're coping. There are good reasons for feeling down, so don't think you're being stupid – and most important of all, don't panic or be afraid.

You might find it useful to:
- write things down in a diary
- make a tape of your favourite music
- go for a walk in the park
- draw or paint.

TALKING TO SOMEONE

It might not always feel that easy, but talking to someone can really help. Friends and family are a good starting point, but if you don't feel comfortable doing this then there are other options.

If you speak to a **doctor**, they should be understanding and offer you advice. Sometimes doctors prescribe tablets, which can be helpful if you're feeling really down, but they can also refer you to a specialist

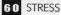

who is trained to help young people deal with problems. Everything you say will be confidential – they won't tell anyone else what you've told them.

If you speak to a **counsellor** or a **therapist** they will also be very sympathetic. They will give you time to think about what you are going through. They are trained, and used to talking to people who have all sorts of worries. And if you're nervous, there's no reason why you can't take a friend with you.

Change takes time and practice – there are no fast cures. Feeling low isn't easy to deal with and stress can turn into depression if you don't deal with your feelings at the outset. You might find ways of coping that give you immediate relief, like drinking or taking drugs for example, but as the next chapter outlines these will end up giving you more problems than answers.

CHAPTER NINE:

DEPENDENCY AND ADDICTION
Alcohol and drugs

Feeling low isn't easy to deal with. And these days there many reasons why we're feeling more and more stressed.

'The pace of life is faster than ever now. There is academic pressure, peer-group pressure to get involved in things like drugs, pressure to find a good job and, for young men especially, our society still expects them to have a stiff upper lip.'

Simon Armson, Chief Executive, Samaritans

You might be tempted to try drugs or drink alcohol because some of your friends want you to, and you don't want to appear different. The pressure to fit in is huge.

But another big reason for teenagers turning to drugs and alcohol is because they think getting drunk or high will help them forget about the stress they're under.

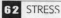

FACT BOX

Boys are ten times more likely to 'self-medicate' in an attempt to beat stress than girls.

It might seem like an instant remedy, but in fact the problems mount up when you start drinking and/or taking drugs as part of your way of coping with stress. In the short term it makes you feel happy, but alcohol is in fact a depressant, making your mood much darker after the initial high.

ALCOHOL

Too much alcohol can:

- **Make you ill**
- **Make you put on weight**
- **Give you a hangover**
- **Cost you a lot of money**
- **Cloud your judgement**
- **Encourage you to do things that are stupid or dangerous**
- **Act as a depressive**

Figure 4 Some effects of alcohol

And there are major concerns that drinking alcohol is becoming a worrying trend amongst teenagers.

FACT BOX

- *Six out of ten boys and half the girls in Year 7 said they had tried at least one alcoholic drink*
- *Eight out of ten students (boys and girls) in Year 11 said they had drunk alcohol in the previous four weeks*
- *According to Alcohol Concern, young people are drinking larger amounts of alcohol and drinking it more often.*

So, if alcohol seems tempting, try to think about the long-term implications. Dependency makes dealing with stress even more of a struggle and what can seem like an easy hit to get rid of all life's worries can in fact add a whole lot more. When you get used to relying on alcohol to make you feel better, it's harder to give it up and find other ways of managing your life.

And the same can be said for drugs. Often regarded as a quick and effective means of relaxing and de-stressing, taking them can give you even more cause for concern.

DRUGS

Drugs, as well as alcohol, might seem an appealing way of de-stressing. After all, you're getting an instant high and all your worries can disappear in an instant. But thinking that you are in control because you're taking just one E or smoking just one spliff, for example, can be deceiving. Getting addicted is a lot easier than you probably realise.

The facts

Different drugs work in different ways. The effects depend on the amount you're doing, where you are and how you're feeling. You might think you're too smart to get addicted, but did you know:

■ As your body gets used to the drug, you need to take more to get the effect you want – meaning that you're increasing the risk of taking an overdose

■ Most people don't realise there's a problem until they're addicted

■ Psychological addiction is a risk with all drugs

■ If drugs appeal as a form of escapism, then dependency is a risk

■ Whether you become addicted can depend on things like your family history, mental state and social situation

■ Physically addictive drugs like tranquillisers, alcohol, sleeping pills and heroin work by changing your body chemistry

■ You can become addicted to any drug that affects your mood, for example cannabis.

What seems like an initial release from all your stresses and worries might seem appealing, but in the long run you'll more than likely end up damaging your body, and your mind too.

> **For a closer look at dependency and addiction,
> see *Real Life Issues: Addictions*.**

Dealing effectively with stress means taking a more holistic approach. That means looking after both your mind and your body. And it's not just therapy for a week or two until you feel better. Learning good coping methods will keep your stress levels at bay throughout your life, whatever the pressures you face.

The following chapter outlines some great ways to de-stress and you can mix and match whichever suit you best.

CHAPTER TEN:

OVERCOMING STRESS
What can I do?

The rule is: if it works for you, it's a good stress-buster. Chilling out is all about individual taste. But some techniques have scientific support for their powers to relieve stress. Here are some things you might not have thought about!

POSITIVE THINKING

The American psychologist Dr Albert Ellis believes that we can teach ourselves to change the way we think, and therefore reduce the amount of stress in our lives. Most stressful events are only stressful because we think they are.

In fact, research published in 2002 in the American Psychological Association's *Journal of Personality and Social Psychology* reveals that optimists tend to have happier lives and are healthier than pessimists, regardless of the degree of stress they experience. And now more and more medics think that helping people to develop healthy ways of thinking is a vital ingredient in any stress management programme.

Many of us who suffer from stress will have what therapists call 'twisted thinking'. This accentuates the negative and can lead us to get more stressed. Here are some examples of twisted thinking:

- You fail to recognise your own accomplishments and achievements, only focusing on what you could have done better.
- You dwell on the negatives and shut out the positives. Maybe nine people will tell you they like what you're wearing. The tenth will tell you they hate your outfit. You'll dwell on the tenth comment.
- You blow everything out of proportion so you feel down more often.
- You're a perfectionist, and that's another key factor that increases stress. Perfectionists can never win since nothing is ever perfect. There is always something, however small, that can be improved.

Training yourself to think differently isn't at all easy but there are some tips that can help:

- Try not to see everything in 'all or nothing' terms – think in small steps.
- Give yourself compliments, like you would your best friend.
- Write down a list of all the good things that have happened to you at the end of the day, or all the things you have achieved, however big or small.

People can become locked into unrealistic thinking patterns. So if you make a mistake, you might automatically feel you're a failure. This is 'twisted thinking', where everything is seen as 'all or nothing' and where problems can be blown out of all proportion. By training your mind to think differently, you can cope with stressful situations much more effectively. Some kinds of therapy can help you with this. You can also make a list of all the positive things you've done.

PLENTY OF PROTEIN

The psychiatrist Dr Hyla Cass recommends getting as much taurine into your system as possible. Taurine is a non-essential amino acid that is thought to calm and stabilise an excited brain by controlling the release of adrenaline. Taurine is highly concentrated in animal and fish protein, but the body also manufactures it from other essential nutrients, so vegetarians shouldn't worry. But it is important to make sure that, even when you are stressed, you are eating a healthy and balanced diet.

FEEL FEMALE

Research by Professor Shelley Taylor, a social psychologist at the University of California, has revealed that men and women respond differently to stress. She found that during the stress response, women release the hormone oxytocin, which encourages them to gather other women around them for support.

Men are less likely to share their feelings because high levels of testosterone inhibit oxytocin's effects. Professor Taylor believes that the female desire to get your friends on board rather than going it alone, as men often do, could be the reason why women live longer than men in developed countries.

So, whether you are male or female, the next time you feel stressed, pick up the phone and call a friend.

STROKE A PET

Dr James Serpell, director of the Center for the Interaction of Animals and Society thinks that domestic animals are the key to a stress-free life. He has shown that just being in the same room as a pet has a calming effect on humans.

SOME USEFUL TIPS

You're not trying to get rid of stressful events in your life – that's impossible. But learning how to cope can help you beat stress. Once you find your own way of coping, you'll realise that it is possible to turn unhealthy stress into healthy pressure. And good stress management is all about learning how to get the most out of life using the least energy.

There are so many different ways in which you can manage your stress levels. Remember to go with whatever feels right for you.

Some of these tips might be a good starting point:
- Learn about stress
- Understand what exactly causes you to be stressed
- Accept that, like everyone else, you have limits
- Eat little and often and don't skip breakfast
- Drink two litres of water a day
- Do more exercise
- Create some leisure time every day
- Make time for friends and family
- Try to laugh at least once a day
- Practise breathing exercises
- Don't put off things you are scared of, as this makes the fear worse – just do it.

TREVOR'S RECIPE FOR A STRESS-FREE LIFE

Trevor Nelson, Radio 1 DJ, has his own recipe for chilling out:

Music
'Your favourite music can alter your mood, pull you through the rough

times in your life and also help you celebrate the better times in your life. Go to live gigs and clubs – there's nothing like the feeling you get after a good shake or dance!'

Sport
'Get active by taking up a new sport. You could try tennis, martial arts or a gym workout. You won't just be getting your body fitter, you'll be doing wonders for your mind too. It's a great way to work off aggression and stress and you'll find you have more energy and better concentration during the day. Getting involved with sport will also help you to meet new people and expand your network of friends.'

Zen baths
'Take a relaxing Zen bath – this is designed to make you focus on your senses. Light a candle, put some smelling salts in your bath and play some relaxing music. Focus on the candlelight for a minute and slowly start to meditate. Try to empty your mind and not to think about anything. It's a great way to unwind at the end of a busy day. Fit in some quiet time in your daily routine. Taking time to relax can help reduce stress.'

Bananas
'Eat a banana! Bananas control serotonin, which is a chemical in the brain that controls self-esteem and optimism, and induces calm feelings. What you eat is closely related to how you're feeling, so eating food that is good for your body will be good for your mind too. You should also try to avoid refined sugar and processed meals, stimulants, caffeine and additives. Instead, opt for plenty of fruit and vegetables and protein-rich foods like fish, meat, milk, eggs, and pulses.'

'A healthy body means a healthy mind.'

Winter blues

'How do you get yourself out of the winter blues – when the clocks have gone back, the nights are drawing in and the weather's getting cold? Get out and about in the daytime – make the most of the daylight by doing an activity. Autumn is a time of seasonal change – maybe now's the time to have a big clearout, or do the thing that you've been meaning to do for ages – like learning to drive. It gives you a sense of achievement and it makes tough times easier to deal with if you have something positive going on in winter months.'

Keep a journal

'If things are getting a bit too much, write down your feelings. It's better than keeping things inside. Getting your innermost feelings down on paper is really liberating and a great way to express yourself. Or, make like Picasso, and get painting! Express your feelings on canvas – it's fun and you get to decorate your bedroom wall with it at the end.'

OTHER METHODS OF GETTING RID OF THAT STRESS

There are many ways to relax and relieve the stress you're under. Some are fairly inexpensive and can do wonders for the way you feel.

Aromatherapy

Aromatherapy uses extracts from plants and trees. These extracts are made into essential oils, which are very strong. They can be used in different ways:

- dilute the oils with water, put them in a burner and inhale them
- sprinkle a few drops on your pillow to help you sleep

- add a few drops of oil to your bath water
- mix essential oils with vegetable oil and massage the mixture into your skin
- lavender helps people to relax and sleep, and can relieve headaches
- patchouli oil reduces anxiety and can help lift your mood
- ylang ylang makes you feel happier and helps you to sleep. But don't use too much, as it can cause headaches.

Books on aromatherapy can tell you which oils to use. Oils can be bought at chemists, health food shops and some high-street stores. You could also see a qualified aromatherapist, although that might be costly.

Martial arts

Martial arts – hand and body movements mostly learned for self-defence – can help relaxation. T'ai chi and aikido are two of the best martial arts for relieving stress and tension.

T'ai chi originates from China and has been practised for thousands of years. It uses body movements and breathing to help clear the mind and body. T'ai chi is also used for self defence.

Aikido originates from Japan. You don't need to be physically strong to practise aikido – quick reactions and flexibility are what count.

Yoga

Yoga helps develop a healthy body and mind. Yoga focuses awareness on your body and the space around you. Tension in your muscles is relaxed and you become more flexible. By focusing attention on your body, your mind can begin to work with a different outlook. In most yoga classes you'll normally spend a few minutes concentrating on your breathing or meditating, then you'll perform stretches which can be performed while lying, standing, or sitting down.

A recent American survey, conducted by the Thomas Jefferson University in Pennsylvania, discovered that after a single session of yoga levels of the stress hormone cortisol dropped, even in people who had never tried yoga before. Cortisol is the hormone that is secreted in the body during stressful times. When we are stressed, cortisol levels increase, and tend to rapidly drop once the stress disappears.

There are several types of yoga including Hatha, Iyengar and Kundalini. Try different styles until you find one that suits you.

Eating your way to a balanced life

And of course, there's that well-known phrase, 'You are what you eat'. It's true. What and how you eat can reflect the way you feel and cope with what life throws at you. Eating properly can help you to look and feel your best! When we talk about a 'balanced diet', we mean that you are eating enough of each different food group in order to give you the nutrients you need for a healthy life.

The Food Guide Pyramid (Figure 5, overleaf) shows you the types of food that make up a good diet. For a balanced diet you need to eat a variety of foods from all five groups. The Food Guide Pyramid tells you how much of the foods from the different groups you should eat to stay healthy.

Its pyramid shape shows which foods you should eat more or less of. The foods that make up the wide base should provide the biggest part

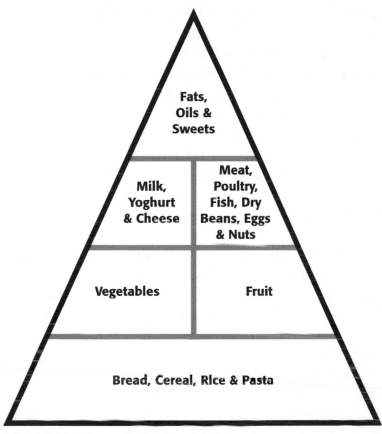

(courtesy kidshealth.com - Nemours Foundation)

Figure 5 The Food Pyramid

of your diet. As you go up the pyramid, the amounts you need get smaller.

BREAD, CEREAL, RICE AND PASTA GROUP

Bread, cereal, rice, and pasta are all great sources of carbohydrate, the nutrient that is the body's major energy provider. So if you're very active and want lots of energy, make sure you have plenty of carbohydrate. This group forms the bottom of the pyramid, so these foods should make up the biggest part of what you eat all day.

VEGETABLE GROUP

Vegetables are great because they are packed full of vitamins and minerals, which are needed to keep your skin, bones and teeth healthy. Carrots are a good source of Vitamin A, and tomatoes are great for Vitamin C. Broccoli and spinach are good, too, because dark green vegetables have more vitamins than lighter vegetables. The vegetable group is towards the bottom of the pyramid because lots of daily servings of vegetables are an important part of a healthy balanced diet.

FRUIT GROUP

Fruits are fantastic because not only to they taste great but they also provide important vitamins that keep you feeling fine and looking good. You will find a lot of Vitamin C in this food group – it's in fruits like oranges, strawberries, watermelon, and lots more. Fruits also give you carbohydrates and fibre. The fruit group is near the bottom of the pyramid, too, so you know daily servings of fruit play a big role in a healthy balanced diet.

MILK, YOGHURT AND CHEESE GROUP

Eating and drinking milk, yoghurt and cheese is the best way to get your daily calcium, which is essential for healthy bones and teeth. There is plenty of protein to help you grow and build your body in this part of the pyramid. This food group is near the top of the pyramid. This means that even though these foods are important for good health, you don't need to eat as many of them in one day as you do of foods further down on the pyramid.

MEAT, POULTRY, FISH, DRY BEANS, EGGS AND NUTS GROUP

This food group is also near the top of the pyramid, again, although important, you don't need to eat as much of them as you do of foods that are lower down on the pyramid. Meat, chicken, fish, beans, eggs, and nuts all supply you with the nutrient protein, which helps you grow. They also provide important minerals iron and zinc.

FATS, OILS AND SWEETS

Fats, oils and sweets sit at the very top of the pyramid, which means that your body should have smaller amounts of them. Your body needs fat for some things, but you should avoid eating too much of it. And although sugary foods like chocolate and biscuits are carbohydrates and can give you an energy boost, they're usually full of calories and don't offer much in the way of nutrients.

The Food Guide Pyramid suggests that when it comes to fatty, oily, or sugary foods, you should consume them less often and in small amounts.

HOW CAN COUNSELLING OR PSYCHOTHERAPY HELP?

There are lots of ways to deal with stress. But if you don't feel you can do it on your own, then perhaps counselling might provide you with the best help. A therapeutic practitioner can help you gain a new way of thinking about whatever is troubling you. Together you identify what's stopping you from reaching your full potential and plan a course of action that will help improve your situation. The aim of the therapeutic process is to help you understand and accept yourself and to change your behaviour to that which is likely to help you become the kind of person you want to be.

Whatever method you choose, it's important to find something that suits you. You might choose a combination of exercise and good eating or decide that counselling is most effective way of helping. What really matters is that you start to identify the feelings of worry and anxiety you have and begin to take control of your feelings. Don't let them get the better of you.

EXAMS

BBC Radio 1's One Life website offers a whole host of revision techniques, what to do about missed exams and the qualifications you need for various jobs. It also contains information and advice about life after exams.

Website: www.bbc.co.uk/radio1/onelife/education

BULLYING

Kidscape

A charity dedicated to preventing bullying. It runs a helpline staffed by trained counsellors. The helpline is available at local rate Monday to Friday from 10am to 4pm. They also offer free confidence-building sessions for children who've been bullied.

Tel: 08451 205204

Website: www.kidscape.org.uk

DEPRESSION

Campaign Against Living Miserably (CALM)

A helpline for 15–24-year-old men experiencing the onset of depression. They give advice, guidance, referrals and counselling.

Website: www.comcarenet.co.uk

Careline

Confidential crisis telephone counselling for children, young people and adults. Careline can refer callers to other organisations and support groups throughout the country.

Tel: 020 8514 1177 (Monday–Friday, 10am–4pm and 7pm–10pm)

Email: careline@totalise.co.uk

Get Connected

Finds young people the best help, whatever the problem. Puts young people in touch with organisations that can help them.

Freephone: 0808 808 4994 (seven days a week, 1pm–11pm)

Website: www.getconnected.org.uk

The Line

Provides free confidential advice, counselling and support for any problem to young people who are living away from home.

Freephone: 0800 884444 (Monday–Friday 3.30pm–9.30pm; weekends 2pm–8pm)

Mental Health Foundation

Has a useful factsheet about depression.

Website: www.mentalhealth.org.uk

MONEY ISSUES

Citizens Advice Bureau (CAB)

Offers free advice about credit and money issues from 700 local bureaux. Search for your nearest CAB online.

Website: www.nacab.org.uk

Consumer Credit Counselling Service (CCCS)

A free and confidential advice service for people in debt. They can help you to prioritise debts and liase with creditors on your behalf.

Wade House

Merrion Centre

Leeds LS2 8NG

Tel: 0800 138 1111

Website: www.cccs.co.uk

Credit Action

National Christian charity, which aims to help people educate themselves about money.

Howard House

The Point

Weaver Road

Lincoln LN6 3QN

Tel: 01522 699777

Website: www.creditaction.org.uk

Email: office@creditaction.org.uk

Department of Social Security

For information on benefits.

Website: www.dss.gov.uk

FCL Debt Clinic

FCL is a free, confidential helpline offering advice and solutions, including supervised arrangements with creditors.

Tel: 0800 716239 (freephone helpline, open Monday–Friday 9am–9pm)

Website: www.fcl.org.uk

Email: help@debtclinic.co.uk

National Debtline

Phone service offering advice and self-help information packs to those in debt.

Tel: 0808 808 4000 (free and confidential)

Website: www.nationaldebtline.co.uk

HOUSING ISSUES

Centrepoint

Provides accommodation, support, training and employment for
16–21-year-olds.

Tel: 020 7287 9134

Housemate

Housing and homelessness information for young people and anyone
who works with young people.

Website: www.housemate.org.uk

Shelter

Information and advice on housing and homelessness.

Tel: 0808 800 4444 (Shelterline, a housing helpline, is open 24
hours a day and is free)

Website: www.shelternet.org.uk

ALCOHOL AND DRUGS

National Association for Children of Alcoholics (NACOA)

The NACOA has a free helpline for young people affected by
alcoholism and lots more advice.

Tel: 01117 924 8005; or freephone 0800 358 3456
(Monday–Friday 9am–5pm)

Website: www.nacoa.org.uk.

Talk to Frank

Free, confidential advice and information about drugs and solvents.
Trained advisors can provide information about local services and give
you support if you are concerned about a drug problem.

Tel: 0800 776600

Website: www.talktofrank.com

RELATIONSHIPS

BBC Health
Lots of information on staying safe and enjoying sex.
Website: www.bbc.co.uk/health/sex/

Relate
Counselling for adults and young people with relationship difficulties.
Little Church Street
Rugby CV21 3AP
Tel: 01788 573241
Website: www.relate.org.uk

LESBIAN, GAY AND BISEXUAL

Avert
AVERT is an AIDS education and medical research charity which also
has information for young people on being gay and coming out.
Website: www.avert.org

Gay-youth-support.com
For anyone who is confused about their sexuality.
Website: www.gay-youth-support.com

Girl Diva
Youth group for lesbian and bisexual women, and those questioning
their sexuality, aged 25 and under.
Website: www.outzone.org/girldiva/intro.htm

PUBERTY

Acne Support Group

Get skin advice online.

Website: www.stopspots.org

BBC Science – Teen Species

A great interactive guide to the way our bodies change during puberty and beyond.

Website: www.bbc.co.uk/science/humanbody

NetDoctor

Try their quiz to find out how good your body image is, and get useful advice on how to deal with negative feelings about your body.

Website: www.netdoctor.co.uk

NHS Direct

Free and confidential health advice and information 24 hours a day, seven days a week, and, most importantly for those potentially sensitive health topics, it can save embarrassment.

Tel: 0845 4647

Website: www.nhsdirect.nhs.uk

Useful publications

Trotman's Real Life Issues series. Self-help books offering information and advice on a range of key issues that matter to you. Each book defines the issue, and offers ways of understanding and coping with it. Real Life Issues aim to demystify the areas that you might find hard to talk about, providing honest facts, practical advice, inspirational quotes and firm reassurance.

Addictions, Stephen Briggs
Confidence and Self-Esteem, Nicki Household
Coping with Life, Jonathan Bradley
Eating Disorders, Heather Warner
Money, Dee Pilgrim
Sex and Relationships, Adele Cherreson
Stress, Rozina Breen